A Life To Be Mindful Network

A LIFE
TO BE
MINDFUL
NETWORK

JENNIFER ALLAN

Matador
Unit E2 Airfield Business Park,
Harrison Road, Market Harborough,
Leicestershire. LE16 7UL
Tel: 0116 279 2299
Email: books@troubador.co.uk
Web: www.troubador.co.uk/matador
Twitter: @matadorbooks

ISBN 9781803135793

British Library Cataloguing in Publication Data.
A catalogue record for this book is available from the British Library.

Printed and bound by CPI Group (UK) Ltd, Croydon, CR0 4YY
Typeset in 12pt Bembo by Troubador Publishing Ltd, Leicester, UK

Matador is an imprint of Troubador Publishing Ltd

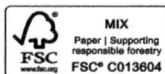

CONTENTS

WELCOME

MANAGING YOUR CIRCUMSTANCES

So what can you do to help with your current circumstances?

Ultimately it starts and ends with you, you just have to recognise that something needs to change. It is the first and hardest step of all, as with most things.

Asking for help isn't failure and should never be viewed as such, asking for help is proof of strength and determination.

Depending on the severity I would always recommend you see your GP, they have lots of great resources and if you both agree, begin on medication.

Counselling is exceptional but can either be too expensive or they have long waiting lists. Speaking with friends or family who understand is a huge help and using this as talking therapy will elliviate such a huge load. Finding yourself a confidant at work or the like can help also as they don't have so much of an investment in you.

Managing your day by establishing a routine, irregardless of whether you have anything specific to do that day is our go to task. Our self help management journal was created for that sole purpose.

Walking in nature, reading a book, going on a course, there are so many things that can assist you…if you are willing to try.

We always recommend breaking down the barriers and feelings one by one. Forget about the mountain ahead, start with the woods at the bottom and chop them down.

Believe you can, and you will. We believe in you.

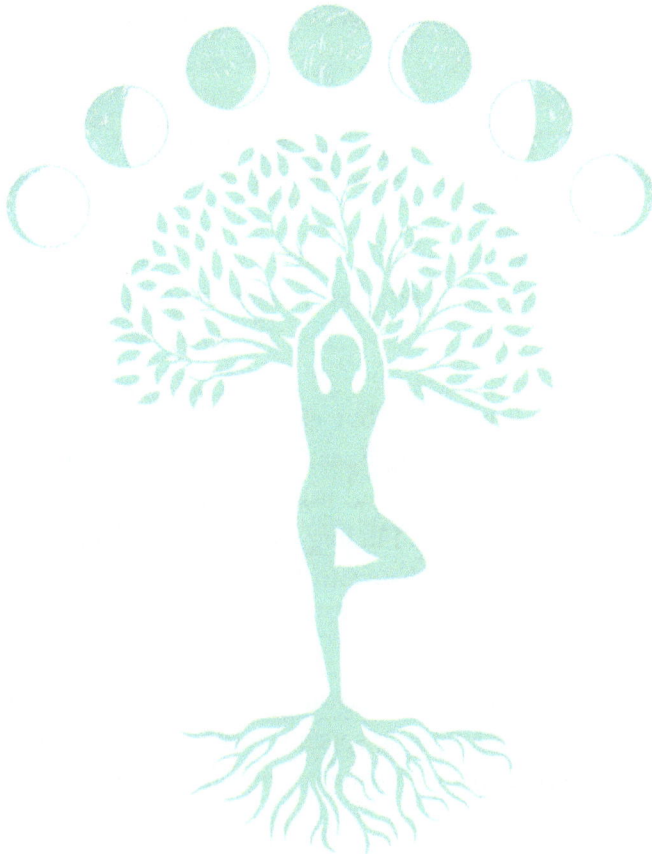

IMBALANCE

When a heaviness creeps into my head
Sometimes it happens getting out of bed.
I look for comfort and a steady hand
Because I feel like I am walking in marsh land.
I'm not angry or sad, I don't even feel mad or bad
I feel nothing for anything.
And nothing within
And I'm not really sure who owns this skin.
Maybe I'll sit and stare at this wall for another day
And hope it keeps my thoughts at bay.
It's a chemical imbalance ignored for so long
Which makes you feel that you don't belong.
Other times with a demon thought
Causes anxiety and feeling distraught.
My reaction is panic and fear
And wanting the world to disappear.
When this turmoil hits you hard
It can still knock you off guard.
Find a friend that will understand
To sit and listen holding your hand.
We are here and think the same
We don't judge or condone, or portion the blame.
Our worth is more not less, this is why I say
On a good day join me, with laughter and play.

Written by John Hyland 2019

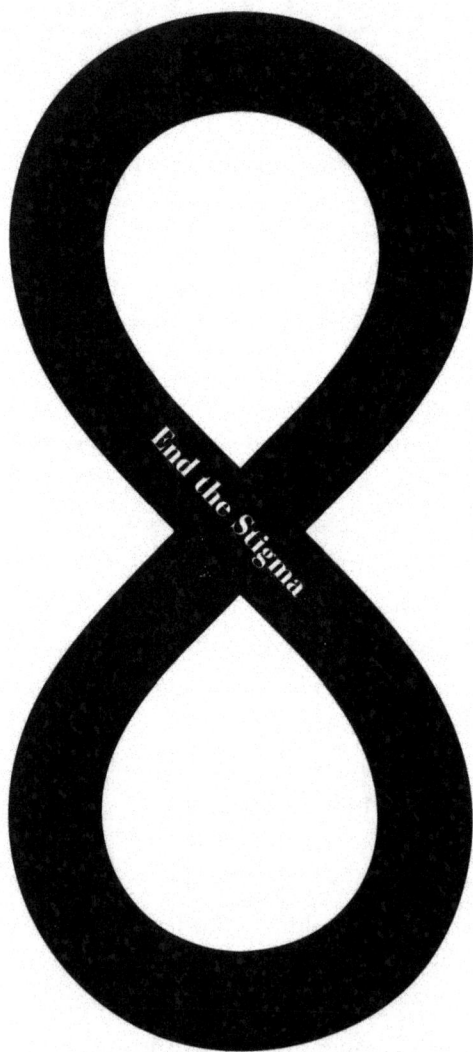

End the Stigma

SEROTONIN

THE FEEL GOOD HORMONE

A naturally occurring transmitter Serotonin is the essential hormone for stabilising your mood and emotional well-being. It also contributes to many vital bodily functions, such as sleep and digestion. Looking out for the symptoms that the levels are unstable is vitally important.

Serotonin is released into the blood stream moving to your Digestive System to communicate signals and stimulate physical reactions.

The Brain needs Serotonin to correctly regulate your moods – maintaining ideal amounts of things like happiness and anxiety. When Serotonin is low it is common to experience depression.

Serotonin affects your sleep, from being able to fall asleep and wakening up. This is why unbalanced Serotonin levels can lead to oversleeping or tiredness based on the lack of sleep.

It is responsible for mood regulation controlling focus, happiness and anxiety.

To increase your Serotonin levels please see your GP, visit the outdoors, focus on your Vitamin D, get moving through exercise and eating Serotonin boosting foods such as oats, whole grain or sweet potatoes.

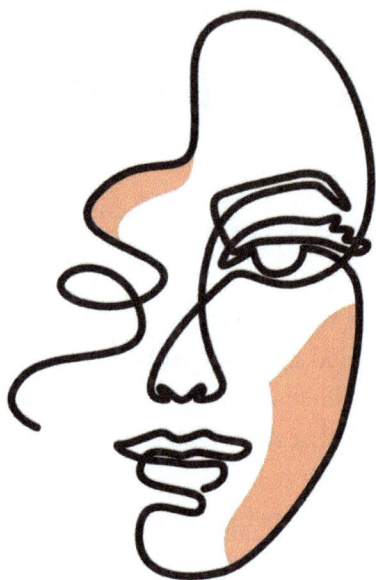

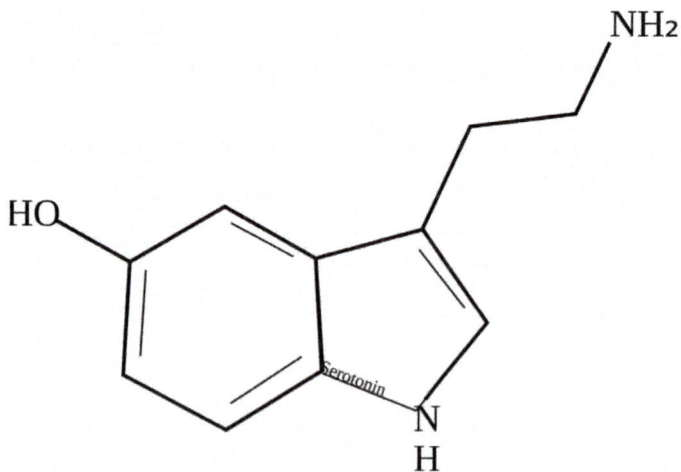

GRATITUDE

WHY BEING GRATEFUL FOR WHAT WE DO HAVE LEAVES POSITIVE IMPRESSIONS ON OUR LIFE.

Everywhere we turn, Social Media, Journals, Television there is always mention of looking & acknowledging our blessings. It has become a 'Trendy' thing to do.

It is something that has become an eye roll scenario, making it a fad. This can be a sore point amongst those who really want to use this method to help you.

SO WHY IS IT IMPORTANT?

Although we see this everywhere it doesn't make it any less effective, but do we ever see an explanation of why it is important to our mindset?

Making the time to list off the things you are grateful for can & will lift the fog/pressure that your mind is under. You may not feel like you have a lot to be thankful for but the few you have is all you need to begin with.

**DAILY REPETITION=HEALTHY HABIT
LIST THEM.
REPEAT THEM.
& REPEAT THEM AGAIN.**

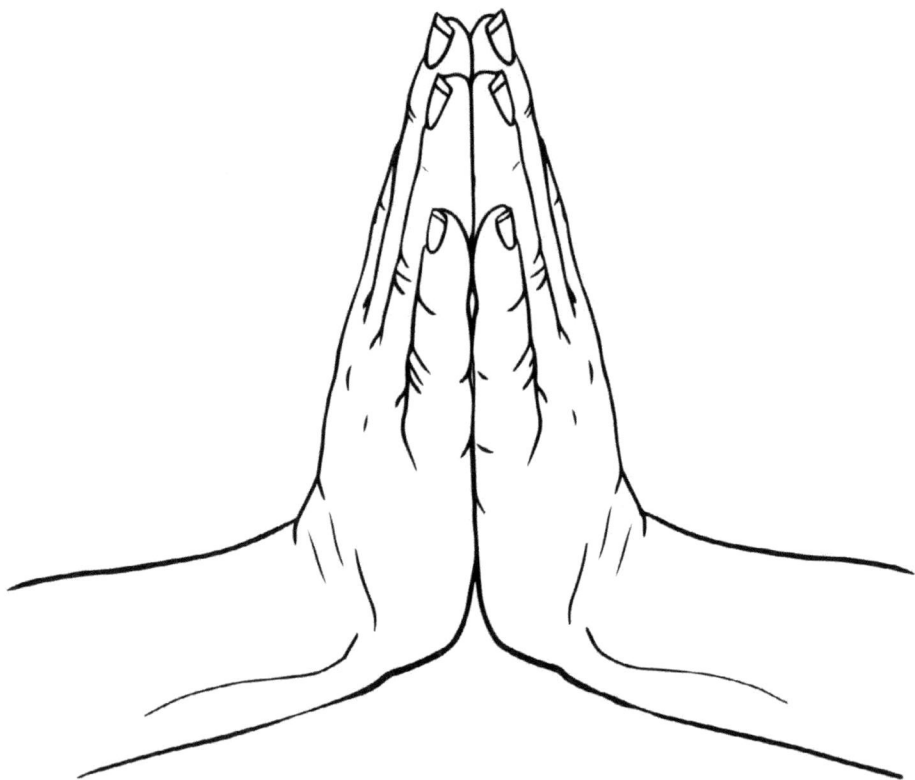

PANIC

How To
Level Out
The Panic:

- Stop what you are doing
- Close your eyes
- Tap your middle right finger as quick as you think your heart rate is
- Start to level out your breathing: in deep through the nose & out through the mouth

Once you feel
that you are
ready:

- Begin to slow the tapping of your finger – the feeling of panic will start to ebb and the calm come over you.
- If you have been bouncing your leg, slow it down – this will come naturally as you steady your tapping.
- Continue to lower the rate of your tapping, right until you're almost at a stop
- Level out your breathing & begin to open your eyes

How do you feel?
How do you feel to be able to control what you thought was uncontrollable?

Puts a smile on your face doesn't it?

Week One

What did today do for you?
Look back on today & reflect. Answer these questions & see what can be do one to make your life more comfortable

Name Three things that you are grateful for today:
Noting the things that we are thankful for starts & ends your day with a happy heart.

_____

_____

_____

_____

Were there any moments of sadness or stress?
And did you do anything to relieve this?

_____

_____

_____

_____

Daily aims
What did you want to achieve today? If you need to, take it into tomorrow

_____

_____

_____

_____

Self Care
It is important to spend at least 10 minutes a day to yourself, what did you do today? Meditate? Walking? Taking a warm Bath?

_____

_____

_____

_____

What are your plans for tomorrow?
Set your intentions for tomorrow now, this will help with
motivation & sleep

_____

_____

_____

_____

Thoughts
This is the time to write down everything that will relieve your
mind. Treat this as your journal

_____

_____

_____

_____

_____

_____

_____

_____

_____

_____

_____

_____

_____

_____

_____

_____

_____

_____

_____

_____

What did today do for you?
Look back on today & reflect. Answer these questions & see
what can be do one to make your life more comfortable

Name Three things that you are grateful for today:
Noting the things that we are thankful for starts & ends your day
with a happy heart.

_____

_____

_____

_____

Were there any moments of sadness or stress?
And did you do anything to relieve this?

_____

_____

_____

_____

Daily aims
What did you want to achieve today? If you need to, take it into
tomorrow

_____

_____

_____

_____

Self Care
It is important to spend at least 10 minutes a day to yourself, what
did you do today? Meditate? Walking? Taking a warm Bath?

_____

_____

_____

_____

What are your plans for tomorrow?
Set your intentions for tomorrow now, this will help with
motivation & sleep

_____

_____

_____

_____

Thoughts
This is the time to write down everything that will relieve your
mind. Treat this as your journal

_____

_____

_____

_____

_____

_____

_____

_____

_____

_____

_____

_____

_____

_____

_____

_____

_____

_____

_____

_____

_____

What did today do for you?
Look back on today & reflect. Answer these questions & see
what can be do one to make your life more comfortable

Name Three things that you are grateful for today:
Noting the things that we are thankful for starts & ends your day
with a happy heart.

_____

_____

_____

_____

Were there any moments of sadness or stress?
And did you do anything to relieve this?

_____

_____

_____

_____

Daily aims
What did you want to achieve today? If you need to, take it into
tomorrow

_____

_____

_____

_____

Self Care
It is important to spend at least 10 minutes a day to yourself, what
did you do today? Meditate? Walking? Taking a warm Bath?

_____

_____

_____

_____

What are your plans for tomorrow?
Set your intentions for tomorrow now, this will help with
motivation & sleep

_____

_____

_____

_____

Thoughts
This is the time to write down everything that will relieve your
mind. Treat this as your journal

_____

_____

_____

_____

_____

_____

_____

_____

_____

_____

_____

_____

_____

_____

_____

_____

_____

_____

_____

_____

_____

What did today do for you?
Look back on today & reflect. Answer these questions & see
what can be do one to make your life more comfortable

Name Three things that you are grateful for today:
Noting the things that we are thankful for starts & ends your day
with a happy heart.

_____

_____

_____

_____

Were there any moments of sadness or stress?
And did you do anything to relieve this?

_____

_____

_____

_____

Daily aims
What did you want to achieve today? If you need to, take it into
tomorrow

_____

_____

_____

_____

Self Care
It is important to spend at least 10 minutes a day to yourself, what
did you do today? Meditate? Walking? Taking a warm Bath?

_____

_____

_____

_____

What are your plans for tomorrow?

Set your intentions for tomorrow now, this will help with
motivation & sleep

_____

_____

_____

_____

Thoughts

This is the time to write down everything that will relieve your
mind. Treat this as your journal

_____

_____

_____

_____

_____

_____

_____

_____

_____

_____

_____

_____

_____

_____

_____

_____

_____

_____

_____

_____

What did today do for you?
Look back on today & reflect. Answer these questions & see
what can be do one to make your life more comfortable

Name Three things that you are grateful for today:
Noting the things that we are thankful for starts & ends your day
with a happy heart.

_____

_____

_____

_____

Were there any moments of sadness or stress?
And did you do anything to relieve this?

_____

_____

_____

_____

Daily aims
What did you want to achieve today? If you need to, take it into
tomorrow

_____

_____

_____

_____

Self Care
It is important to spend at least 10 minutes a day to yourself, what
did you do today? Meditate? Walking? Taking a warm Bath?

_____

_____

_____

_____

What are your plans for tomorrow?
Set your intentions for tomorrow now, this will help with
motivation & sleep

_____

_____

_____

_____

Thoughts
This is the time to write down everything that will relieve your
mind. Treat this as your journal

_____

_____

_____

_____

_____

_____

_____

_____

_____

_____

_____

_____

_____

_____

_____

_____

_____

_____

_____

_____

What did today do for you?

Look back on today & reflect. Answer these questions & see what can be do one to make your life more comfortable

Name Three things that you are grateful for today:

Noting the things that we are thankful for starts & ends your day with a happy heart.

_____

_____

_____

_____

Were there any moments of sadness or stress?

And did you do anything to relieve this?

_____

_____

_____

_____

Daily aims

What did you want to achieve today? If you need to, take it into tomorrow

_____

_____

_____

_____

Self Care

It is important to spend at least 10 minutes a day to yourself, what did you do today? Meditate? Walking? Taking a warm Bath?

_____

_____

_____

_____

What are your plans for tomorrow?

Set your intentions for tomorrow now, this will help with
motivation & sleep

_____

_____

_____

_____

Thoughts

This is the time to write down everything that will relieve your
mind. Treat this as your journal

_____

_____

_____

_____

_____

_____

_____

_____

_____

_____

_____

_____

_____

_____

_____

_____

_____

_____

_____

What did today do for you?
Look back on today & reflect. Answer these questions & see
what can be do one to make your life more comfortable

Name Three things that you are grateful for today:
Noting the things that we are thankful for starts & ends your day
with a happy heart.

_____

_____

_____

_____

Were there any moments of sadness or stress?
And did you do anything to relieve this?

_____

_____

_____

_____

Daily aims
What did you want to achieve today? If you need to, take it into
tomorrow

_____

_____

_____

_____

Self Care
It is important to spend at least 10 minutes a day to yourself, what
did you do today? Meditate? Walking? Taking a warm Bath?

_____

_____

_____

_____

What are your plans for tomorrow?
Set your intentions for tomorrow now, this will help with
motivation & sleep

_____

_____

_____

_____

Thoughts
This is the time to write down everything that will relieve your
mind. Treat this as your journal

_____

_____

_____

_____

_____

_____

_____

_____

_____

_____

_____

_____

_____

_____

_____

_____

_____

_____

_____

_____

Weekly Reflection

Now is the time to look back on your week & reflect. What worked best for you? What will you take into next week & continue with? Note below as you would a list.

What decisions have you come to, to make your day easier?

_____

_____

_____

_____

What were your highs & lows?

_____

_____

_____

_____

What would you like to tackle next week?

_____

_____

_____

_____

WELL DONE ON A SUCCESSFUL WEEK! Whether you believe it or not trying is a success in itself!

KEEP GOING! You are worth your determination

Week Two

What did today do for you?
Look back on today & reflect. Answer these questions & see
what can be do one to make your life more comfortable

Name Three things that you are grateful for today:
Noting the things that we are thankful for starts & ends your day
with a happy heart.

_____
_____
_____
_____

Were there any moments of sadness or stress?
And did you do anything to relieve this?

_____
_____
_____
_____

Daily aims
What did you want to achieve today? If you need to, take it into
tomorrow

_____
_____
_____
_____

Self Care
It is important to spend at least 10 minutes a day to yourself, what
did you do today? Meditate? Walking? Taking a warm Bath?

_____
_____
_____
_____

What are your plans for tomorrow?
Set your intentions for tomorrow now, this will help with
motivation & sleep

_____

_____

_____

_____

Thoughts
This is the time to write down everything that will relieve your
mind. Treat this as your journal

_____

_____

_____

_____

_____

_____

_____

_____

_____

_____

_____

_____

_____

_____

_____

_____

_____

_____

What did today do for you?
Look back on today & reflect. Answer these questions & see
what can be do one to make your life more comfortable

Name Three things that you are grateful for today:
Noting the things that we are thankful for starts & ends your day
with a happy heart.

_____

_____

_____

_____

Were there any moments of sadness or stress?
And did you do anything to relieve this?

_____

_____

_____

Daily aims
What did you want to achieve today? If you need to, take it into
tomorrow

_____

_____

_____

_____

Self Care
It is important to spend at least 10 minutes a day to yourself, what
did you do today? Meditate? Walking? Taking a warm Bath?

_____

_____

_____

_____

What are your plans for tomorrow?
Set your intentions for tomorrow now, this will help with
motivation & sleep

_____

_____

_____

_____

Thoughts
This is the time to write down everything that will relieve your
mind. Treat this as your journal

_____

_____

_____

_____

_____

_____

_____

_____

_____

_____

_____

_____

_____

_____

_____

_____

_____

_____

_____

_____

_____

What did today do for you?
Look back on today & reflect. Answer these questions & see what can be do one to make your life more comfortable

Name Three things that you are grateful for today:
Noting the things that we are thankful for starts & ends your day with a happy heart.

_____

_____

_____

_____

Were there any moments of sadness or stress?
And did you do anything to relieve this?

_____

_____

_____

_____

Daily aims
What did you want to achieve today? If you need to, take it into tomorrow

_____

_____

_____

_____

Self Care
It is important to spend at least 10 minutes a day to yourself, what did you do today? Meditate? Walking? Taking a warm Bath?

_____

_____

_____

_____

What are your plans for tomorrow?
Set your intentions for tomorrow now, this will help with
motivation & sleep

Thoughts
This is the time to write down everything that will relieve your
mind. Treat this as your journal

What did today do for you?

Look back on today & reflect. Answer these questions & see what can be do one to make your life more comfortable

Name Three things that you are grateful for today:

Noting the things that we are thankful for starts & ends your day with a happy heart.

_____

_____

_____

_____

Were there any moments of sadness or stress?

And did you do anything to relieve this?

_____

_____

_____

_____

Daily aims

What did you want to achieve today? If you need to, take it into tomorrow

_____

_____

_____

_____

Self Care

It is important to spend at least 10 minutes a day to yourself, what did you do today? Meditate? Walking? Taking a warm Bath?

_____

_____

_____

_____

What are your plans for tomorrow?
Set your intentions for tomorrow now, this will help with
motivation & sleep

_____

_____

_____

_____

Thoughts
This is the time to write down everything that will relieve your
mind. Treat this as your journal

_____

_____

_____

_____

_____

_____

_____

_____

_____

_____

_____

_____

_____

_____

_____

_____

_____

_____

_____

_____

_____

_____

_____

What did today do for you?

Look back on today & reflect. Answer these questions & see what can be do one to make your life more comfortable

Name Three things that you are grateful for today:

Noting the things that we are thankful for starts & ends your day with a happy heart.

_____

_____

_____

_____

Were there any moments of sadness or stress?

And did you do anything to relieve this?

_____

_____

_____

_____

Daily aims

What did you want to achieve today? If you need to, take it into tomorrow

_____

_____

_____

_____

Self Care

It is important to spend at least 10 minutes a day to yourself, what did you do today? Meditate? Walking? Taking a warm Bath?

_____

_____

_____

_____

What are your plans for tomorrow?
Set your intentions for tomorrow now, this will help with
motivation & sleep

_____

_____

_____

_____

Thoughts
This is the time to write down everything that will relieve your
mind. Treat this as your journal

_____

_____

_____

_____

_____

_____

_____

_____

_____

_____

_____

_____

_____

_____

_____

_____

_____

_____

_____

_____

What did today do for you?

Look back on today & reflect. Answer these questions & see what can be do one to make your life more comfortable

Name Three things that you are grateful for today:

Noting the things that we are thankful for starts & ends your day with a happy heart.

_____

_____

_____

_____

Were there any moments of sadness or stress?

And did you do anything to relieve this?

_____

_____

_____

_____

Daily aims

What did you want to achieve today? If you need to, take it into tomorrow

_____

_____

_____

_____

Self Care

It is important to spend at least 10 minutes a day to yourself, what did you do today? Meditate? Walking? Taking a warm Bath?

_____

_____

_____

_____

What are your plans for tomorrow?
Set your intentions for tomorrow now, this will help with motivation & sleep

_____

_____

_____

_____

Thoughts
This is the time to write down everything that will relieve your mind. Treat this as your journal

_____

_____

_____

_____

_____

_____

_____

_____

_____

_____

_____

_____

_____

_____

_____

_____

_____

_____

_____

_____

_____

_____

What did today do for you?

Look back on today & reflect. Answer these questions & see what can be do one to make your life more comfortable

Name Three things that you are grateful for today:

Noting the things that we are thankful for starts & ends your day with a happy heart.

_____

_____

_____

_____

Were there any moments of sadness or stress?

And did you do anything to relieve this?

_____

_____

_____

_____

Daily aims

What did you want to achieve today? If you need to, take it into tomorrow

_____

_____

_____

_____

Self Care

It is important to spend at least 10 minutes a day to yourself, what did you do today? Meditate? Walking? Taking a warm Bath?

_____

_____

_____

_____

What are your plans for tomorrow?
Set your intentions for tomorrow now, this will help with motivation & sleep

_____

_____

_____

_____

Thoughts
This is the time to write down everything that will relieve your mind. Treat this as your journal

_____

_____

_____

_____

_____

_____

_____

_____

_____

_____

_____

_____

_____

_____

_____

_____

_____

_____

_____

_____

_____

_____

Weekly Reflection

Now is the time to look back on your week & reflect. What worked best for you? What will you take into next week & continue with? Note below as you would a list.

What decisions have you come to, to make your day easier?

_____

_____

_____

_____

What were your highs & lows?

_____

_____

_____

_____

What would you like to tackle next week?

_____

_____

_____

_____

WELL DONE ON A SUCCESSFUL WEEK! Whether you believe it or not trying is a success in itself!

KEEP GOING! You are worth your determination

Week Three

What did today do for you?
Look back on today & reflect. Answer these questions & see
what can be do one to make your life more comfortable

Name Three things that you are grateful for today:
Noting the things that we are thankful for starts & ends your day
with a happy heart.

_____

_____

_____

_____

Were there any moments of sadness or stress?
And did you do anything to relieve this?

_____

_____

_____

_____

Daily aims
What did you want to achieve today? If you need to, take it into
tomorrow

_____

_____

_____

_____

Self Care
It is important to spend at least 10 minutes a day to yourself, what
did you do today? Meditate? Walking? Taking a warm Bath?

_____

_____

_____

_____

What are your plans for tomorrow?
Set your intentions for tomorrow now, this will help with
motivation & sleep

_____

_____

_____

_____

Thoughts
This is the time to write down everything that will relieve your
mind. Treat this as your journal

_____

_____

_____

_____

_____

_____

_____

_____

_____

_____

_____

_____

_____

_____

_____

_____

_____

_____

_____

_____

_____

_____

_____

What did today do for you?

Look back on today & reflect. Answer these questions & see what can be do one to make your life more comfortable

Name Three things that you are grateful for today:

Noting the things that we are thankful for starts & ends your day with a happy heart.

_____

_____

_____

_____

Were there any moments of sadness or stress?

And did you do anything to relieve this?

_____

_____

_____

_____

Daily aims

What did you want to achieve today? If you need to, take it into tomorrow

_____

_____

_____

_____

Self Care

It is important to spend at least 10 minutes a day to yourself, what did you do today? Meditate? Walking? Taking a warm Bath?

_____

_____

_____

_____

What are your plans for tomorrow?
Set your intentions for tomorrow now, this will help with
motivation & sleep

_____

_____

_____

_____

Thoughts
This is the time to write down everything that will relieve your
mind. Treat this as your journal

_____

_____

_____

_____

_____

_____

_____

_____

_____

_____

_____

_____

_____

_____

_____

_____

_____

_____

_____

_____

_____

What did today do for you?
Look back on today & reflect. Answer these questions & see
what can be do one to make your life more comfortable

Name Three things that you are grateful for today:
Noting the things that we are thankful for starts & ends your day
with a happy heart.

_____

_____

_____

_____

Were there any moments of sadness or stress?
And did you do anything to relieve this?

_____

_____

_____

_____

Daily aims
What did you want to achieve today? If you need to, take it into
tomorrow

_____

_____

_____

_____

Self Care
It is important to spend at least 10 minutes a day to yourself, what
did you do today? Meditate? Walking? Taking a warm Bath?

_____

_____

_____

_____

What are your plans for tomorrow?
Set your intentions for tomorrow now, this will help with
motivation & sleep

_____

_____

_____

_____

Thoughts
This is the time to write down everything that will relieve your
mind. Treat this as your journal

_____

_____

_____

_____

_____

_____

_____

_____

_____

_____

_____

_____

_____

_____

_____

_____

_____

_____

_____

_____

What did today do for you?

Look back on today & reflect. Answer these questions & see what can be do one to make your life more comfortable

Name Three things that you are grateful for today:

Noting the things that we are thankful for starts & ends your day with a happy heart.

_____

_____

_____

_____

Were there any moments of sadness or stress?

And did you do anything to relieve this?

_____

_____

_____

_____

Daily aims

What did you want to achieve today? If you need to, take it into tomorrow

_____

_____

_____

_____

Self Care

It is important to spend at least 10 minutes a day to yourself, what did you do today? Meditate? Walking? Taking a warm Bath?

_____

_____

_____

_____

What are your plans for tomorrow?
Set your intentions for tomorrow now, this will help with
motivation & sleep

_____

_____

_____

_____

Thoughts
This is the time to write down everything that will relieve your
mind. Treat this as your journal

_____

_____

_____

_____

_____

_____

_____

_____

_____

_____

_____

_____

_____

_____

_____

_____

_____

_____

_____

_____

_____

_____

What did today do for you?

Look back on today & reflect. Answer these questions & see what can be do one to make your life more comfortable

Name Three things that you are grateful for today:

Noting the things that we are thankful for starts & ends your day with a happy heart.

_____

_____

_____

_____

Were there any moments of sadness or stress?

And did you do anything to relieve this?

_____

_____

_____

_____

Daily aims

What did you want to achieve today? If you need to, take it into tomorrow

_____

_____

_____

_____

Self Care

It is important to spend at least 10 minutes a day to yourself, what did you do today? Meditate? Walking? Taking a warm Bath?

_____

_____

_____

_____

What are your plans for tomorrow?
Set your intentions for tomorrow now, this will help with
motivation & sleep

_____

_____

_____

_____

Thoughts
This is the time to write down everything that will relieve your
mind. Treat this as your journal

_____

_____

_____

_____

_____

_____

_____

_____

_____

_____

_____

_____

_____

_____

_____

_____

_____

_____

_____

_____

_____

What did today do for you?
Look back on today & reflect. Answer these questions & see
what can be do one to make your life more comfortable

Name Three things that you are grateful for today:
Noting the things that we are thankful for starts & ends your day
with a happy heart.

_____

_____

_____

_____

Were there any moments of sadness or stress?
And did you do anything to relieve this?

_____

_____

_____

_____

Daily aims
What did you want to achieve today? If you need to, take it into
tomorrow

_____

_____

_____

_____

Self Care
It is important to spend at least 10 minutes a day to yourself, what
did you do today? Meditate? Walking? Taking a warm Bath?

_____

_____

_____

_____

What are your plans for tomorrow?
Set your intentions for tomorrow now, this will help with
motivation & sleep

_____

_____

_____

_____

Thoughts
This is the time to write down everything that will relieve your
mind. Treat this as your journal

_____

_____

_____

_____

_____

_____

_____

_____

_____

_____

_____

_____

_____

_____

_____

_____

_____

_____

_____

_____

_____

_____

What did today do for you?

Look back on today & reflect. Answer these questions & see what can be do one to make your life more comfortable

Name Three things that you are grateful for today:

Noting the things that we are thankful for starts & ends your day with a happy heart.

_____

_____

_____

_____

Were there any moments of sadness or stress?

And did you do anything to relieve this?

_____

_____

_____

_____

Daily aims

What did you want to achieve today? If you need to, take it into tomorrow

_____

_____

_____

_____

Self Care

It is important to spend at least 10 minutes a day to yourself, what did you do today? Meditate? Walking? Taking a warm Bath?

_____

_____

_____

_____

What are your plans for tomorrow?
Set your intentions for tomorrow now, this will help with
motivation & sleep

_____

_____

_____

_____

Thoughts
This is the time to write down everything that will relieve your
mind. Treat this as your journal

_____

_____

_____

_____

_____

_____

_____

_____

_____

_____

_____

_____

_____

_____

_____

_____

_____

_____

_____

_____

Weekly Reflection

Now is the time to look back on your week & reflect. What worked best for you? What will you take into next week & continue with? Note below as you would a list.

What decisions have you come to, to make your day easier?

_____

_____

_____

_____

What were your highs & lows?

_____

_____

_____

_____

What would you like to tackle next week?

_____

_____

_____

_____

WELL DONE ON A SUCCESSFUL WEEK! Whether you believe it or not trying is a success in itself!

KEEP GOING! You are worth your determination

Week Four

What did today do for you?

Look back on today & reflect. Answer these questions & see what can be do one to make your life more comfortable

Name Three things that you are grateful for today:

Noting the things that we are thankful for starts & ends your day with a happy heart.

_____

_____

_____

_____

Were there any moments of sadness or stress?

And did you do anything to relieve this?

_____

_____

_____

_____

Daily aims

What did you want to achieve today? If you need to, take it into tomorrow

_____

_____

_____

_____

Self Care

It is important to spend at least 10 minutes a day to yourself, what did you do today? Meditate? Walking? Taking a warm Bath?

_____

_____

_____

_____

What are your plans for tomorrow?
Set your intentions for tomorrow now, this will help with motivation & sleep

_____

_____

_____

_____

Thoughts
This is the time to write down everything that will relieve your mind. Treat this as your journal

What did today do for you?
Look back on today & reflect. Answer these questions & see
what can be do one to make your life more comfortable

Name Three things that you are grateful for today:
Noting the things that we are thankful for starts & ends your day
with a happy heart.

_____

_____

_____

_____

Were there any moments of sadness or stress?
And did you do anything to relieve this?

_____

_____

_____

_____

Daily aims
What did you want to achieve today? If you need to, take it into
tomorrow

_____

_____

_____

_____

Self Care
It is important to spend at least 10 minutes a day to yourself, what
did you do today? Meditate? Walking? Taking a warm Bath?

_____

_____

_____

_____

What are your plans for tomorrow?
Set your intentions for tomorrow now, this will help with
motivation & sleep

_____

_____

_____

_____

Thoughts
This is the time to write down everything that will relieve your
mind. Treat this as your journal

_____

_____

_____

_____

_____

_____

_____

_____

_____

_____

_____

_____

_____

_____

_____

_____

_____

_____

_____

_____

_____

What did today do for you?
Look back on today & reflect. Answer these questions & see
what can be do one to make your life more comfortable

Name Three things that you are grateful for today:
Noting the things that we are thankful for starts & ends your day
with a happy heart.

_____

_____

_____

_____

Were there any moments of sadness or stress?
And did you do anything to relieve this?

_____

_____

_____

_____

Daily aims
What did you want to achieve today? If you need to, take it into
tomorrow

_____

_____

_____

_____

Self Care
It is important to spend at least 10 minutes a day to yourself, what
did you do today? Meditate? Walking? Taking a warm Bath?

_____

_____

_____

_____

What are your plans for tomorrow?
Set your intentions for tomorrow now, this will help with
motivation & sleep

_____

_____

_____

_____

Thoughts
This is the time to write down everything that will relieve your
mind. Treat this as your journal

_____

_____

_____

_____

_____

_____

_____

_____

_____

_____

_____

_____

_____

_____

_____

_____

_____

_____

_____

_____

_____

_____

What did today do for you?
Look back on today & reflect. Answer these questions & see
what can be do one to make your life more comfortable

Name Three things that you are grateful for today:
Noting the things that we are thankful for starts & ends your day
with a happy heart.

_____

_____

_____

_____

Were there any moments of sadness or stress?
And did you do anything to relieve this?

_____

_____

_____

_____

Daily aims
What did you want to achieve today? If you need to, take it into
tomorrow

_____

_____

_____

_____

Self Care
It is important to spend at least 10 minutes a day to yourself, what
did you do today? Meditate? Walking? Taking a warm Bath?

_____

_____

_____

_____

What are your plans for tomorrow?
Set your intentions for tomorrow now, this will help with motivation & sleep

_____

_____

_____

_____

Thoughts
This is the time to write down everything that will relieve your mind. Treat this as your journal

_____

_____

_____

_____

_____

_____

_____

_____

_____

_____

_____

_____

_____

_____

_____

_____

_____

_____

_____

_____

_____

_____

What did today do for you?
Look back on today & reflect. Answer these questions & see
what can be do one to make your life more comfortable

Name Three things that you are grateful for today:
Noting the things that we are thankful for starts & ends your day
with a happy heart.

_____

_____

_____

_____

Were there any moments of sadness or stress?
And did you do anything to relieve this?

_____

_____

_____

_____

Daily aims
What did you want to achieve today? If you need to, take it into
tomorrow

_____

_____

_____

_____

Self Care
It is important to spend at least 10 minutes a day to yourself, what
did you do today? Meditate? Walking? Taking a warm Bath?

_____

_____

_____

_____

What are your plans for tomorrow?
Set your intentions for tomorrow now, this will help with
motivation & sleep

_____

_____

_____

_____

Thoughts
This is the time to write down everything that will relieve your
mind. Treat this as your journal

_____

_____

_____

_____

_____

_____

_____

_____

_____

_____

_____

_____

_____

_____

_____

_____

_____

_____

_____

_____

What did today do for you?
Look back on today & reflect. Answer these questions & see what can be do one to make your life more comfortable

Name Three things that you are grateful for today:
Noting the things that we are thankful for starts & ends your day with a happy heart.

_____

_____

_____

_____

Were there any moments of sadness or stress?
And did you do anything to relieve this?

_____

_____

_____

_____

Daily aims
What did you want to achieve today? If you need to, take it into tomorrow

_____

_____

_____

_____

Self Care
It is important to spend at least 10 minutes a day to yourself, what did you do today? Meditate? Walking? Taking a warm Bath?

_____

_____

_____

_____

What are your plans for tomorrow?
Set your intentions for tomorrow now, this will help with
motivation & sleep

Thoughts
This is the time to write down everything that will relieve your
mind. Treat this as your journal

What did today do for you?
Look back on today & reflect. Answer these questions & see
what can be do one to make your life more comfortable

Name Three things that you are grateful for today:
Noting the things that we are thankful for starts & ends your day
with a happy heart.

_____

_____

_____

_____

Were there any moments of sadness or stress?
And did you do anything to relieve this?

_____

_____

_____

_____

Daily aims
What did you want to achieve today? If you need to, take it into
tomorrow

_____

_____

_____

_____

Self Care
It is important to spend at least 10 minutes a day to yourself, what
did you do today? Meditate? Walking? Taking a warm Bath?

_____

_____

_____

_____

What are your plans for tomorrow?
Set your intentions for tomorrow now, this will help with
motivation & sleep

_____

_____

_____

_____

Thoughts
This is the time to write down everything that will relieve your
mind. Treat this as your journal

_____

_____

_____

_____

_____

_____

_____

_____

_____

_____

_____

_____

_____

_____

_____

_____

_____

_____

_____

_____

Weekly Reflection

Now is the time to look back on your week & reflect. What worked best for you? What will you take into next week & continue with? Note below as you would a list.

What decisions have you come to, to make your day easier?

_____

_____

_____

_____

What were your highs & lows?

_____

_____

_____

_____

What would you like to tackle next week?

_____

_____

_____

_____

WELL DONE ON A SUCCESSFUL WEEK! Whether you believe it or not trying is a success in itself!

KEEP GOING! You are worth your determination

Week Five

What did today do for you?
Look back on today & reflect. Answer these questions & see what can be do one to make your life more comfortable

Name Three things that you are grateful for today:
Noting the things that we are thankful for starts & ends your day with a happy heart.

_____

_____

_____

_____

Were there any moments of sadness or stress?
And did you do anything to relieve this?

_____

_____

_____

_____

Daily aims
What did you want to achieve today? If you need to, take it into tomorrow

_____

_____

_____

_____

Self Care
It is important to spend at least 10 minutes a day to yourself, what did you do today? Meditate? Walking? Taking a warm Bath?

_____

_____

_____

_____

What are your plans for tomorrow?
Set your intentions for tomorrow now, this will help with
motivation & sleep

_____

_____

_____

_____

Thoughts
This is the time to write down everything that will relieve your
mind. Treat this as your journal

_____

_____

_____

_____

_____

_____

_____

_____

_____

_____

_____

_____

_____

_____

_____

_____

_____

_____

_____

_____

What did today do for you?
Look back on today & reflect. Answer these questions & see
what can be do one to make your life more comfortable

Name Three things that you are grateful for today:
Noting the things that we are thankful for starts & ends your day
with a happy heart.

_____

_____

_____

_____

Were there any moments of sadness or stress?
And did you do anything to relieve this?

_____

_____

_____

_____

Daily aims
What did you want to achieve today? If you need to, take it into
tomorrow

_____

_____

_____

_____

Self Care
It is important to spend at least 10 minutes a day to yourself, what
did you do today? Meditate? Walking? Taking a warm Bath?

_____

_____

_____

_____

What are your plans for tomorrow?
Set your intentions for tomorrow now, this will help with
motivation & sleep

_____

_____

_____

_____

Thoughts
This is the time to write down everything that will relieve your
mind. Treat this as your journal

_____

_____

_____

_____

_____

_____

_____

_____

_____

_____

_____

_____

_____

_____

_____

_____

_____

_____

_____

_____

_____

What did today do for you?

Look back on today & reflect. Answer these questions & see what can be do one to make your life more comfortable

Name Three things that you are grateful for today:

Noting the things that we are thankful for starts & ends your day with a happy heart.

_____

_____

_____

_____

Were there any moments of sadness or stress?

And did you do anything to relieve this?

_____

_____

_____

_____

Daily aims

What did you want to achieve today? If you need to, take it into tomorrow

_____

_____

_____

_____

Self Care

It is important to spend at least 10 minutes a day to yourself, what did you do today? Meditate? Walking? Taking a warm Bath?

_____

_____

_____

_____

What are your plans for tomorrow?
Set your intentions for tomorrow now, this will help with motivation & sleep

_____

_____

_____

_____

Thoughts
This is the time to write down everything that will relieve your mind. Treat this as your journal

_____

_____

_____

_____

_____

_____

_____

_____

_____

_____

_____

_____

_____

_____

_____

_____

_____

_____

_____

What did today do for you?
Look back on today & reflect. Answer these questions & see
what can be do one to make your life more comfortable

Name Three things that you are grateful for today:
Noting the things that we are thankful for starts & ends your day
with a happy heart.

_____

_____

_____

_____

Were there any moments of sadness or stress?
And did you do anything to relieve this?

_____

_____

_____

_____

Daily aims
What did you want to achieve today? If you need to, take it into
tomorrow

_____

_____

_____

_____

Self Care
It is important to spend at least 10 minutes a day to yourself, what
did you do today? Meditate? Walking? Taking a warm Bath?

_____

_____

_____

_____

What are your plans for tomorrow?
Set your intentions for tomorrow now, this will help with
motivation & sleep

_____

_____

_____

_____

Thoughts
This is the time to write down everything that will relieve your
mind. Treat this as your journal

_____

_____

_____

_____

_____

_____

_____

_____

_____

_____

_____

_____

_____

_____

_____

_____

_____

_____

_____

_____

_____

What did today do for you?

Look back on today & reflect. Answer these questions & see
what can be do one to make your life more comfortable

Name Three things that you are grateful for today:

Noting the things that we are thankful for starts & ends your day
with a happy heart.

_____

_____

_____

_____

Were there any moments of sadness or stress?

And did you do anything to relieve this?

_____

_____

_____

_____

Daily aims

What did you want to achieve today? If you need to, take it into
tomorrow

_____

_____

_____

_____

Self Care

It is important to spend at least 10 minutes a day to yourself, what
did you do today? Meditate? Walking? Taking a warm Bath?

_____

_____

_____

_____

What are your plans for tomorrow?
Set your intentions for tomorrow now, this will help with
motivation & sleep

_____

_____

_____

_____

Thoughts
This is the time to write down everything that will relieve your
mind. Treat this as your journal

_____

_____

_____

_____

_____

_____

_____

_____

_____

_____

_____

_____

_____

_____

_____

_____

_____

_____

_____

_____

What did today do for you?
Look back on today & reflect. Answer these questions & see what can be do one to make your life more comfortable

Name Three things that you are grateful for today:
Noting the things that we are thankful for starts & ends your day with a happy heart.

_____

_____

_____

_____

Were there any moments of sadness or stress?
And did you do anything to relieve this?

_____

_____

_____

_____

Daily aims
What did you want to achieve today? If you need to, take it into tomorrow

_____

_____

_____

_____

Self Care
It is important to spend at least 10 minutes a day to yourself, what did you do today? Meditate? Walking? Taking a warm Bath?

_____

_____

_____

_____

What are your plans for tomorrow?
Set your intentions for tomorrow now, this will help with
motivation & sleep

_____

_____

_____

_____

Thoughts
This is the time to write down everything that will relieve your
mind. Treat this as your journal

_____

_____

_____

_____

_____

_____

_____

_____

_____

_____

_____

_____

_____

_____

_____

_____

_____

_____

_____

_____

_____

What did today do for you?
Look back on today & reflect. Answer these questions & see what can be do one to make your life more comfortable

Name Three things that you are grateful for today:
Noting the things that we are thankful for starts & ends your day with a happy heart.

_____

_____

_____

_____

Were there any moments of sadness or stress?
And did you do anything to relieve this?

_____

_____

_____

_____

Daily aims
What did you want to achieve today? If you need to, take it into tomorrow

_____

_____

_____

_____

Self Care
It is important to spend at least 10 minutes a day to yourself, what did you do today? Meditate? Walking? Taking a warm Bath?

_____

_____

_____

_____

What are your plans for tomorrow?
Set your intentions for tomorrow now, this will help with motivation & sleep

_____

_____

_____

_____

Thoughts
This is the time to write down everything that will relieve your mind. Treat this as your journal

_____

_____

_____

_____

_____

_____

_____

_____

_____

_____

_____

_____

_____

_____

_____

_____

_____

_____

_____

_____

Weekly Reflection

Now is the time to look back on your week & reflect. What worked best for you? What will you take into next week & continue with? Note below as you would a list.

What decisions have you come to, to make your day easier?

_____

_____

_____

_____

What were your highs & lows?

_____

_____

_____

_____

What would you like to tackle next week?

_____

_____

_____

_____

WELL DONE ON A SUCCESSFUL WEEK! Whether you believe it or not trying is a success in itself!

KEEP GOING! You are worth your determination

Week Six

What did today do for you?

Look back on today & reflect. Answer these questions & see what can be do one to make your life more comfortable

Name Three things that you are grateful for today:

Noting the things that we are thankful for starts & ends your day with a happy heart.

_____

_____

_____

_____

Were there any moments of sadness or stress?

And did you do anything to relieve this?

_____

_____

_____

_____

Daily aims

What did you want to achieve today? If you need to, take it into tomorrow

_____

_____

_____

_____

Self Care

It is important to spend at least 10 minutes a day to yourself, what did you do today? Meditate? Walking? Taking a warm Bath?

_____

_____

_____

_____

What are your plans for tomorrow?
Set your intentions for tomorrow now, this will help with
motivation & sleep

_____

_____

_____

_____

Thoughts
This is the time to write down everything that will relieve your
mind. Treat this as your journal

_____

_____

_____

_____

_____

_____

_____

_____

_____

_____

_____

_____

_____

_____

_____

_____

_____

_____

_____

_____

What did today do for you?
Look back on today & reflect. Answer these questions & see
what can be do one to make your life more comfortable

Name Three things that you are grateful for today:
Noting the things that we are thankful for starts & ends your day
with a happy heart.

_____

_____

_____

_____

Were there any moments of sadness or stress?
And did you do anything to relieve this?

_____

_____

_____

_____

Daily aims
What did you want to achieve today? If you need to, take it into
tomorrow

_____

_____

_____

_____

Self Care
It is important to spend at least 10 minutes a day to yourself, what
did you do today? Meditate? Walking? Taking a warm Bath?

_____

_____

_____

_____

What are your plans for tomorrow?
Set your intentions for tomorrow now, this will help with
motivation & sleep

_____

_____

_____

_____

Thoughts
This is the time to write down everything that will relieve your
mind. Treat this as your journal

_____

_____

_____

_____

_____

_____

_____

_____

_____

_____

_____

_____

_____

_____

_____

_____

_____

_____

_____

_____

_____

_____

What did today do for you?

Look back on today & reflect. Answer these questions & see
what can be do one to make your life more comfortable

Name Three things that you are grateful for today:

Noting the things that we are thankful for starts & ends your day
with a happy heart.

_____

_____

_____

_____

Were there any moments of sadness or stress?

And did you do anything to relieve this?

_____

_____

_____

_____

Daily aims

What did you want to achieve today? If you need to, take it into
tomorrow

_____

_____

_____

_____

Self Care

It is important to spend at least 10 minutes a day to yourself, what
did you do today? Meditate? Walking? Taking a warm Bath?

_____

_____

_____

_____

What are your plans for tomorrow?
Set your intentions for tomorrow now, this will help with
motivation & sleep

_____

_____

_____

_____

Thoughts
This is the time to write down everything that will relieve your
mind. Treat this as your journal

_____

_____

_____

_____

_____

_____

_____

_____

_____

_____

_____

_____

_____

_____

_____

_____

_____

_____

_____

_____

_____

What did today do for you?
Look back on today & reflect. Answer these questions & see what can be do one to make your life more comfortable

Name Three things that you are grateful for today:
Noting the things that we are thankful for starts & ends your day with a happy heart.

_____

_____

_____

_____

Were there any moments of sadness or stress?
And did you do anything to relieve this?

_____

_____

_____

_____

Daily aims
What did you want to achieve today? If you need to, take it into tomorrow

_____

_____

_____

_____

Self Care
It is important to spend at least 10 minutes a day to yourself, what did you do today? Meditate? Walking? Taking a warm Bath?

_____

_____

_____

_____

What are your plans for tomorrow?
Set your intentions for tomorrow now, this will help with
motivation & sleep

_____

_____

_____

_____

Thoughts
This is the time to write down everything that will relieve your
mind. Treat this as your journal

_____

_____

_____

_____

_____

_____

_____

_____

_____

_____

_____

_____

_____

_____

_____

_____

_____

_____

_____

_____

_____

What did today do for you?
Look back on today & reflect. Answer these questions & see what can be do one to make your life more comfortable

Name Three things that you are grateful for today:
Noting the things that we are thankful for starts & ends your day with a happy heart.

_____

_____

_____

_____

Were there any moments of sadness or stress?
And did you do anything to relieve this?

_____

_____

_____

_____

Daily aims
What did you want to achieve today? If you need to, take it into tomorrow

_____

_____

_____

_____

Self Care
It is important to spend at least 10 minutes a day to yourself, what did you do today? Meditate? Walking? Taking a warm Bath?

_____

_____

_____

_____

What are your plans for tomorrow?
Set your intentions for tomorrow now, this will help with motivation & sleep

_____

_____

_____

_____

Thoughts
This is the time to write down everything that will relieve your mind. Treat this as your journal

_____

_____

_____

_____

_____

_____

_____

_____

_____

_____

_____

_____

_____

_____

_____

_____

_____

_____

_____

What did today do for you?
Look back on today & reflect. Answer these questions & see what can be do one to make your life more comfortable

Name Three things that you are grateful for today:
Noting the things that we are thankful for starts & ends your day with a happy heart.

_____

_____

_____

_____

Were there any moments of sadness or stress?
And did you do anything to relieve this?

_____

_____

_____

_____

Daily aims
What did you want to achieve today? If you need to, take it into tomorrow

_____

_____

_____

_____

Self Care
It is important to spend at least 10 minutes a day to yourself, what did you do today? Meditate? Walking? Taking a warm Bath?

_____

_____

_____

_____

What are your plans for tomorrow?
Set your intentions for tomorrow now, this will help with motivation & sleep

_____

_____

_____

_____

Thoughts
This is the time to write down everything that will relieve your mind. Treat this as your journal

_____

_____

_____

_____

_____

_____

_____

_____

_____

_____

_____

_____

_____

_____

_____

_____

_____

_____

_____

_____

What did today do for you?
Look back on today & reflect. Answer these questions & see what can be do one to make your life more comfortable

Name Three things that you are grateful for today:
Noting the things that we are thankful for starts & ends your day with a happy heart.

_____

_____

_____

_____

Were there any moments of sadness or stress?
And did you do anything to relieve this?

_____

_____

_____

_____

Daily aims
What did you want to achieve today? If you need to, take it into tomorrow

_____

_____

_____

_____

Self Care
It is important to spend at least 10 minutes a day to yourself, what did you do today? Meditate? Walking? Taking a warm Bath?

_____

_____

_____

_____

What are your plans for tomorrow?
Set your intentions for tomorrow now, this will help with
motivation & sleep

_____

_____

_____

_____

Thoughts
This is the time to write down everything that will relieve your
mind. Treat this as your journal

_____

_____

_____

_____

_____

_____

_____

_____

_____

_____

_____

_____

_____

_____

_____

_____

_____

_____

_____

_____

Weekly Reflection

Now is the time to look back on your week & reflect. What worked best for you? What will you take into next week & continue with? Note below as you would a list.

What decisions have you come to, to make your day easier?

_____

_____

_____

_____

What were your highs & lows?

_____

_____

_____

_____

What would you like to tackle next week?

_____

_____

_____

_____

WELL DONE ON A SUCCESSFUL WEEK! Whether you believe it or not trying is a success in itself!

KEEP GOING! You are worth your determination

Week Seven

What did today do for you?
Look back on today & reflect. Answer these questions & see
what can be do one to make your life more comfortable

Name Three things that you are grateful for today:
Noting the things that we are thankful for starts & ends your day
with a happy heart.

_____

_____

_____

_____

Were there any moments of sadness or stress?
And did you do anything to relieve this?

_____

_____

_____

_____

Daily aims
What did you want to achieve today? If you need to, take it into
tomorrow

_____

_____

_____

_____

Self Care
It is important to spend at least 10 minutes a day to yourself, what
did you do today? Meditate? Walking? Taking a warm Bath?

_____

_____

_____

_____

What are your plans for tomorrow?

Set your intentions for tomorrow now, this will help with motivation & sleep

_____

_____

_____

_____

Thoughts

This is the time to write down everything that will relieve your mind. Treat this as your journal

_____

_____

_____

_____

_____

_____

_____

_____

_____

_____

_____

_____

_____

_____

_____

_____

_____

_____

_____

What did today do for you?

Look back on today & reflect. Answer these questions & see
what can be do one to make your life more comfortable

Name Three things that you are grateful for today:

Noting the things that we are thankful for starts & ends your day
with a happy heart.

_____

_____

_____

_____

Were there any moments of sadness or stress?

And did you do anything to relieve this?

_____

_____

_____

_____

Daily aims

What did you want to achieve today? If you need to, take it into
tomorrow

_____

_____

_____

_____

Self Care

It is important to spend at least 10 minutes a day to yourself, what
did you do today? Meditate? Walking? Taking a warm Bath?

_____

_____

_____

_____

What are your plans for tomorrow?
Set your intentions for tomorrow now, this will help with
motivation & sleep

_____

_____

_____

_____

Thoughts
This is the time to write down everything that will relieve your
mind. Treat this as your journal

_____

_____

_____

_____

_____

_____

_____

_____

_____

_____

_____

_____

_____

_____

_____

_____

_____

_____

_____

_____

_____

_____

What did today do for you?

Look back on today & reflect. Answer these questions & see
what can be do one to make your life more comfortable

Name Three things that you are grateful for today:

Noting the things that we are thankful for starts & ends your day
with a happy heart.

_____

_____

_____

_____

Were there any moments of sadness or stress?

And did you do anything to relieve this?

_____

_____

_____

_____

Daily aims

What did you want to achieve today? If you need to, take it into
tomorrow

_____

_____

_____

_____

Self Care

It is important to spend at least 10 minutes a day to yourself, what
did you do today? Meditate? Walking? Taking a warm Bath?

_____

_____

_____

_____

What are your plans for tomorrow?
Set your intentions for tomorrow now, this will help with
motivation & sleep

_____

_____

_____

_____

Thoughts
This is the time to write down everything that will relieve your
mind. Treat this as your journal

_____

_____

_____

_____

_____

_____

_____

_____

_____

_____

_____

_____

_____

_____

_____

_____

_____

_____

_____

_____

What did today do for you?
Look back on today & reflect. Answer these questions & see what can be do one to make your life more comfortable

Name Three things that you are grateful for today:
Noting the things that we are thankful for starts & ends your day with a happy heart.

_____
_____
_____
_____

Were there any moments of sadness or stress?
And did you do anything to relieve this?

_____
_____
_____
_____

Daily aims
What did you want to achieve today? If you need to, take it into tomorrow

_____
_____
_____
_____

Self Care
It is important to spend at least 10 minutes a day to yourself, what did you do today? Meditate? Walking? Taking a warm Bath?

_____
_____
_____
_____

What are your plans for tomorrow?

Set your intentions for tomorrow now, this will help with motivation & sleep

_____

_____

_____

_____

Thoughts

This is the time to write down everything that will relieve your mind. Treat this as your journal

_____

_____

_____

_____

_____

_____

_____

_____

_____

_____

_____

_____

_____

_____

_____

_____

_____

_____

_____

_____

What did today do for you?
Look back on today & reflect. Answer these questions & see what can be do one to make your life more comfortable

Name Three things that you are grateful for today:
Noting the things that we are thankful for starts & ends your day with a happy heart.

_____

_____

_____

_____

Were there any moments of sadness or stress?
And did you do anything to relieve this?

_____

_____

_____

_____

Daily aims
What did you want to achieve today? If you need to, take it into tomorrow

_____

_____

_____

_____

Self Care
It is important to spend at least 10 minutes a day to yourself, what did you do today? Meditate? Walking? Taking a warm Bath?

_____

_____

_____

_____

What are your plans for tomorrow?
Set your intentions for tomorrow now, this will help with motivation & sleep

_____

_____

_____

_____

Thoughts
This is the time to write down everything that will relieve your mind. Treat this as your journal

_____

_____

_____

_____

_____

_____

_____

_____

_____

_____

_____

_____

_____

_____

_____

_____

_____

_____

_____

What did today do for you?

Look back on today & reflect. Answer these questions & see what can be do one to make your life more comfortable

Name Three things that you are grateful for today:

Noting the things that we are thankful for starts & ends your day with a happy heart.

_____

_____

_____

_____

Were there any moments of sadness or stress?

And did you do anything to relieve this?

_____

_____

_____

_____

Daily aims

What did you want to achieve today? If you need to, take it into tomorrow

_____

_____

_____

_____

Self Care

It is important to spend at least 10 minutes a day to yourself, what did you do today? Meditate? Walking? Taking a warm Bath?

_____

_____

_____

_____

What are your plans for tomorrow?
Set your intentions for tomorrow now, this will help with
motivation & sleep

_____

_____

_____

_____

Thoughts
This is the time to write down everything that will relieve your
mind. Treat this as your journal

_____

_____

_____

_____

_____

_____

_____

_____

_____

_____

_____

_____

_____

_____

_____

_____

_____

_____

_____

_____

_____

What did today do for you?

Look back on today & reflect. Answer these questions & see what can be do one to make your life more comfortable

Name Three things that you are grateful for today:

Noting the things that we are thankful for starts & ends your day with a happy heart.

_____

_____

_____

_____

Were there any moments of sadness or stress?

And did you do anything to relieve this?

_____

_____

_____

_____

Daily aims

What did you want to achieve today? If you need to, take it into tomorrow

_____

_____

_____

_____

Self Care

It is important to spend at least 10 minutes a day to yourself, what did you do today? Meditate? Walking? Taking a warm Bath?

_____

_____

_____

_____

What are your plans for tomorrow?
Set your intentions for tomorrow now, this will help with motivation & sleep

_____

_____

_____

_____

Thoughts
This is the time to write down everything that will relieve your mind. Treat this as your journal

_____

_____

_____

_____

_____

_____

_____

_____

_____

_____

_____

_____

_____

_____

_____

_____

_____

_____

_____

Weekly Reflection

Now is the time to look back on your week & reflect. What worked best for you? What will you take into next week & continue with? Note below as you would a list.

What decisions have you come to, to make your day easier?

_____

_____

_____

_____

What were your highs & lows?

_____

_____

_____

_____

What would you like to tackle next week?

_____

_____

_____

_____

WELL DONE ON A SUCCESSFUL WEEK! Whether you believe it or not trying is a success in itself!

KEEP GOING! You are worth your determination

Week Eight

What did today do for you?

Look back on today & reflect. Answer these questions & see
what can be do one to make your life more comfortable

Name Three things that you are grateful for today:

Noting the things that we are thankful for starts & ends your day
with a happy heart.

_____

_____

_____

_____

Were there any moments of sadness or stress?

And did you do anything to relieve this?

_____

_____

_____

_____

Daily aims

What did you want to achieve today? If you need to, take it into
tomorrow

_____

_____

_____

_____

Self Care

It is important to spend at least 10 minutes a day to yourself, what
did you do today? Meditate? Walking? Taking a warm Bath?

_____

_____

_____

_____

What are your plans for tomorrow?
Set your intentions for tomorrow now, this will help with
motivation & sleep

_____

_____

_____

_____

Thoughts
This is the time to write down everything that will relieve your
mind. Treat this as your journal

_____

_____

_____

_____

_____

_____

_____

_____

_____

_____

_____

_____

_____

_____

_____

_____

_____

_____

_____

_____

_____

_____

_____

What did today do for you?
Look back on today & reflect. Answer these questions & see
what can be do one to make your life more comfortable

Name Three things that you are grateful for today:
Noting the things that we are thankful for starts & ends your day
with a happy heart.

_____

_____

_____

_____

Were there any moments of sadness or stress?
And did you do anything to relieve this?

_____

_____

_____

_____

Daily aims
What did you want to achieve today? If you need to, take it into
tomorrow

_____

_____

_____

_____

Self Care
It is important to spend at least 10 minutes a day to yourself, what
did you do today? Meditate? Walking? Taking a warm Bath?

_____

_____

_____

_____

What are your plans for tomorrow?
Set your intentions for tomorrow now, this will help with motivation & sleep

_____

_____

_____

_____

Thoughts
This is the time to write down everything that will relieve your mind. Treat this as your journal

_____

_____

_____

_____

_____

_____

_____

_____

_____

_____

_____

_____

_____

_____

_____

_____

_____

_____

_____

_____

What did today do for you?

Look back on today & reflect. Answer these questions & see what can be do one to make your life more comfortable

Name Three things that you are grateful for today:

Noting the things that we are thankful for starts & ends your day with a happy heart.

_____

_____

_____

_____

Were there any moments of sadness or stress?

And did you do anything to relieve this?

_____

_____

_____

_____

Daily aims

What did you want to achieve today? If you need to, take it into tomorrow

_____

_____

_____

_____

Self Care

It is important to spend at least 10 minutes a day to yourself, what did you do today? Meditate? Walking? Taking a warm Bath?

_____

_____

_____

_____

What are your plans for tomorrow?
Set your intentions for tomorrow now, this will help with
motivation & sleep

_____

_____

_____

_____

Thoughts
This is the time to write down everything that will relieve your
mind. Treat this as your journal

_____

_____

_____

_____

_____

_____

_____

_____

_____

_____

_____

_____

_____

_____

_____

_____

_____

_____

_____

_____

_____

What did today do for you?

Look back on today & reflect. Answer these questions & see
what can be do one to make your life more comfortable

Name Three things that you are grateful for today:

Noting the things that we are thankful for starts & ends your day
with a happy heart.

_____

_____

_____

_____

Were there any moments of sadness or stress?

And did you do anything to relieve this?

_____

_____

_____

_____

Daily aims

What did you want to achieve today? If you need to, take it into
tomorrow

_____

_____

_____

_____

Self Care

It is important to spend at least 10 minutes a day to yourself, what
did you do today? Meditate? Walking? Taking a warm Bath?

_____

_____

_____

_____

What are your plans for tomorrow?
Set your intentions for tomorrow now, this will help with motivation & sleep

_____

_____

_____

_____

Thoughts
This is the time to write down everything that will relieve your mind. Treat this as your journal

_____

_____

_____

_____

_____

_____

_____

_____

_____

_____

_____

_____

_____

_____

_____

_____

_____

_____

_____

_____

_____

What did today do for you?

Look back on today & reflect. Answer these questions & see what can be do one to make your life more comfortable

Name Three things that you are grateful for today:

Noting the things that we are thankful for starts & ends your day with a happy heart.

_____

_____

_____

_____

Were there any moments of sadness or stress?

And did you do anything to relieve this?

_____

_____

_____

_____

Daily aims

What did you want to achieve today? If you need to, take it into tomorrow

_____

_____

_____

_____

Self Care

It is important to spend at least 10 minutes a day to yourself, what did you do today? Meditate? Walking? Taking a warm Bath?

_____

_____

_____

_____

What are your plans for tomorrow?
Set your intentions for tomorrow now, this will help with
motivation & sleep

_____

_____

_____

_____

Thoughts
This is the time to write down everything that will relieve your
mind. Treat this as your journal

_____

_____

_____

_____

_____

_____

_____

_____

_____

_____

_____

_____

_____

_____

_____

_____

_____

_____

_____

_____

_____

What did today do for you?
Look back on today & reflect. Answer these questions & see what can be do one to make your life more comfortable

Name Three things that you are grateful for today:
Noting the things that we are thankful for starts & ends your day with a happy heart.

_____

_____

_____

_____

Were there any moments of sadness or stress?
And did you do anything to relieve this?

_____

_____

_____

_____

Daily aims
What did you want to achieve today? If you need to, take it into tomorrow

_____

_____

_____

_____

Self Care
It is important to spend at least 10 minutes a day to yourself, what did you do today? Meditate? Walking? Taking a warm Bath?

_____

_____

_____

_____

What are your plans for tomorrow?
Set your intentions for tomorrow now, this will help with
motivation & sleep

_____

_____

_____

_____

Thoughts
This is the time to write down everything that will relieve your
mind. Treat this as your journal

_____

_____

_____

_____

_____

_____

_____

_____

_____

_____

_____

_____

_____

_____

_____

_____

_____

_____

_____

_____

What did today do for you?
Look back on today & reflect. Answer these questions & see
what can be do one to make your life more comfortable

Name Three things that you are grateful for today:
Noting the things that we are thankful for starts & ends your day
with a happy heart.

_____

_____

_____

_____

Were there any moments of sadness or stress?
And did you do anything to relieve this?

_____

_____

_____

_____

Daily aims
What did you want to achieve today? If you need to, take it into
tomorrow

_____

_____

_____

_____

Self Care
It is important to spend at least 10 minutes a day to yourself, what
did you do today? Meditate? Walking? Taking a warm Bath?

_____

_____

_____

_____

What are your plans for tomorrow?
Set your intentions for tomorrow now, this will help with motivation & sleep

_____

_____

_____

_____

Thoughts
This is the time to write down everything that will relieve your mind. Treat this as your journal

_____

_____

_____

_____

_____

_____

_____

_____

_____

_____

_____

_____

_____

_____

_____

_____

_____

_____

_____

_____

Weekly Reflection

Now is the time to look back on your week & reflect. What worked best for you? What will you take into next week & continue with? Note below as you would a list.

What decisions have you come to, to make your day easier?

_____

_____

_____

_____

What were your highs & lows?

_____

_____

_____

_____

What would you like to tackle next week?

_____

_____

_____

_____

WELL DONE ON A SUCCESSFUL WEEK! Whether you believe it or not trying is a success in itself!

KEEP GOING! You are worth your determination

Week Nine

What did today do for you?

Look back on today & reflect. Answer these questions & see what can be do one to make your life more comfortable

Name Three things that you are grateful for today:

Noting the things that we are thankful for starts & ends your day with a happy heart.

_____

_____

_____

_____

Were there any moments of sadness or stress?

And did you do anything to relieve this?

_____

_____

_____

_____

Daily aims

What did you want to achieve today? If you need to, take it into tomorrow

_____

_____

_____

_____

Self Care

It is important to spend at least 10 minutes a day to yourself, what did you do today? Meditate? Walking? Taking a warm Bath?

_____

_____

_____

_____

What are your plans for tomorrow?
Set your intentions for tomorrow now, this will help with
motivation & sleep

_____

_____

_____

_____

Thoughts
This is the time to write down everything that will relieve your
mind. Treat this as your journal

_____

_____

_____

_____

_____

_____

_____

_____

_____

_____

_____

_____

_____

_____

_____

_____

_____

_____

_____

_____

_____

What did today do for you?

Look back on today & reflect. Answer these questions & see what can be do one to make your life more comfortable

Name Three things that you are grateful for today:

Noting the things that we are thankful for starts & ends your day with a happy heart.

_____

_____

_____

_____

Were there any moments of sadness or stress?

And did you do anything to relieve this?

_____

_____

_____

_____

Daily aims

What did you want to achieve today? If you need to, take it into tomorrow

_____

_____

_____

_____

Self Care

It is important to spend at least 10 minutes a day to yourself, what did you do today? Meditate? Walking? Taking a warm Bath?

_____

_____

_____

_____

What are your plans for tomorrow?
Set your intentions for tomorrow now, this will help with
motivation & sleep

_____

_____

_____

_____

Thoughts
This is the time to write down everything that will relieve your
mind. Treat this as your journal

_____

_____

_____

_____

_____

_____

_____

_____

_____

_____

_____

_____

_____

_____

_____

_____

_____

_____

_____

_____

What did today do for you?
Look back on today & reflect. Answer these questions & see
what can be do one to make your life more comfortable

Name Three things that you are grateful for today:
Noting the things that we are thankful for starts & ends your day
with a happy heart.

_____
_____
_____
_____

Were there any moments of sadness or stress?
And did you do anything to relieve this?

_____
_____
_____
_____

Daily aims
What did you want to achieve today? If you need to, take it into
tomorrow

_____
_____
_____
_____

Self Care
It is important to spend at least 10 minutes a day to yourself, what
did you do today? Meditate? Walking? Taking a warm Bath?

_____
_____
_____
_____

What are your plans for tomorrow?
Set your intentions for tomorrow now, this will help with
motivation & sleep

_____

_____

_____

_____

Thoughts
This is the time to write down everything that will relieve your
mind. Treat this as your journal

_____

_____

_____

_____

_____

_____

_____

_____

_____

_____

_____

_____

_____

_____

_____

_____

_____

_____

_____

_____

_____

What did today do for you?
Look back on today & reflect. Answer these questions & see what can be do one to make your life more comfortable

Name Three things that you are grateful for today:
Noting the things that we are thankful for starts & ends your day with a happy heart.

_____

_____

_____

_____

Were there any moments of sadness or stress?
And did you do anything to relieve this?

_____

_____

_____

_____

Daily aims
What did you want to achieve today? If you need to, take it into tomorrow

_____

_____

_____

_____

Self Care
It is important to spend at least 10 minutes a day to yourself, what did you do today? Meditate? Walking? Taking a warm Bath?

_____

_____

_____

_____

What are your plans for tomorrow?
Set your intentions for tomorrow now, this will help with motivation & sleep

---

Thoughts
This is the time to write down everything that will relieve your mind. Treat this as your journal

---

What did today do for you?

Look back on today & reflect. Answer these questions & see what can be do one to make your life more comfortable

Name Three things that you are grateful for today:

Noting the things that we are thankful for starts & ends your day with a happy heart.

_____

_____

_____

_____

Were there any moments of sadness or stress?

And did you do anything to relieve this?

_____

_____

_____

_____

Daily aims

What did you want to achieve today? If you need to, take it into tomorrow

_____

_____

_____

_____

Self Care

It is important to spend at least 10 minutes a day to yourself, what did you do today? Meditate? Walking? Taking a warm Bath?

_____

_____

_____

_____

What are your plans for tomorrow?
Set your intentions for tomorrow now, this will help with motivation & sleep

_____

_____

_____

_____

Thoughts
This is the time to write down everything that will relieve your mind. Treat this as your journal

_____

_____

_____

_____

_____

_____

_____

_____

_____

_____

_____

_____

_____

_____

_____

_____

_____

_____

_____

What did today do for you?

Look back on today & reflect. Answer these questions & see what can be do one to make your life more comfortable

Name Three things that you are grateful for today:

Noting the things that we are thankful for starts & ends your day with a happy heart.

_____

_____

_____

_____

Were there any moments of sadness or stress?

And did you do anything to relieve this?

_____

_____

_____

_____

Daily aims

What did you want to achieve today? If you need to, take it into tomorrow

_____

_____

_____

_____

Self Care

It is important to spend at least 10 minutes a day to yourself, what did you do today? Meditate? Walking? Taking a warm Bath?

_____

_____

_____

_____

What are your plans for tomorrow?
Set your intentions for tomorrow now, this will help with
motivation & sleep

Thoughts
This is the time to write down everything that will relieve your
mind. Treat this as your journal

What did today do for you?
Look back on today & reflect. Answer these questions & see
what can be do one to make your life more comfortable

Name Three things that you are grateful for today:
Noting the things that we are thankful for starts & ends your day
with a happy heart.

_____

_____

_____

_____

Were there any moments of sadness or stress?
And did you do anything to relieve this?

_____

_____

_____

_____

Daily aims
What did you want to achieve today? If you need to, take it into
tomorrow

_____

_____

_____

_____

Self Care
It is important to spend at least 10 minutes a day to yourself, what
did you do today? Meditate? Walking? Taking a warm Bath?

_____

_____

_____

_____

What are your plans for tomorrow?
Set your intentions for tomorrow now, this will help with
motivation & sleep

_____

_____

_____

_____

Thoughts
This is the time to write down everything that will relieve your
mind. Treat this as your journal

_____

_____

_____

_____

_____

_____

_____

_____

_____

_____

_____

_____

_____

_____

_____

_____

_____

_____

_____

_____

_____

_____

Weekly Reflection

Now is the time to look back on your week & reflect. What
worked best for you? What will you take into next week &
continue with? Note below as you would a list.

**What decisions have you come to, to make your day
easier?**

_____

_____

_____

_____

What were your highs & lows?

_____

_____

_____

_____

What would you like to tackle next week?

_____

_____

_____

_____

WELL DONE ON A SUCCESSFUL WEEK! Whether you
believe it or not trying is a success in itself!

KEEP GOING! You are worth your determination

Week Ten

What did today do for you?

Look back on today & reflect. Answer these questions & see what can be do one to make your life more comfortable

Name Three things that you are grateful for today:

Noting the things that we are thankful for starts & ends your day with a happy heart.

_____

_____

_____

_____

Were there any moments of sadness or stress?

And did you do anything to relieve this?

_____

_____

_____

_____

Daily aims

What did you want to achieve today? If you need to, take it into tomorrow

_____

_____

_____

_____

Self Care

It is important to spend at least 10 minutes a day to yourself, what did you do today? Meditate? Walking? Taking a warm Bath?

_____

_____

_____

_____

What are your plans for tomorrow?
Set your intentions for tomorrow now, this will help with
motivation & sleep

Thoughts
This is the time to write down everything that will relieve your
mind. Treat this as your journal

What did today do for you?
Look back on today & reflect. Answer these questions & see what can be do one to make your life more comfortable

Name Three things that you are grateful for today:
Noting the things that we are thankful for starts & ends your day with a happy heart.

_____

_____

_____

_____

Were there any moments of sadness or stress?
And did you do anything to relieve this?

_____

_____

_____

Daily aims
What did you want to achieve today? If you need to, take it into tomorrow

_____

_____

_____

_____

Self Care
It is important to spend at least 10 minutes a day to yourself, what did you do today? Meditate? Walking? Taking a warm Bath?

_____

_____

_____

_____

What are your plans for tomorrow?
Set your intentions for tomorrow now, this will help with
motivation & sleep

Thoughts
This is the time to write down everything that will relieve your
mind. Treat this as your journal

What did today do for you?
Look back on today & reflect. Answer these questions & see
what can be do one to make your life more comfortable

Name Three things that you are grateful for today:
Noting the things that we are thankful for starts & ends your day
with a happy heart.

_____

_____

_____

_____

Were there any moments of sadness or stress?
And did you do anything to relieve this?

_____

_____

_____

_____

Daily aims
What did you want to achieve today? If you need to, take it into
tomorrow

_____

_____

_____

_____

Self Care
It is important to spend at least 10 minutes a day to yourself, what
did you do today? Meditate? Walking? Taking a warm Bath?

_____

_____

_____

_____

What are your plans for tomorrow?
Set your intentions for tomorrow now, this will help with
motivation & sleep

_____

_____

_____

_____

Thoughts
This is the time to write down everything that will relieve your
mind. Treat this as your journal

_____

_____

_____

_____

_____

_____

_____

_____

_____

_____

_____

_____

_____

_____

_____

_____

_____

_____

_____

_____

What did today do for you?
Look back on today & reflect. Answer these questions & see what can be do one to make your life more comfortable

Name Three things that you are grateful for today:
Noting the things that we are thankful for starts & ends your day with a happy heart.

_____

_____

_____

_____

Were there any moments of sadness or stress?
And did you do anything to relieve this?

_____

_____

_____

_____

Daily aims
What did you want to achieve today? If you need to, take it into tomorrow

_____

_____

_____

_____

Self Care
It is important to spend at least 10 minutes a day to yourself, what did you do today? Meditate? Walking? Taking a warm Bath?

_____

_____

_____

_____

What are your plans for tomorrow?
Set your intentions for tomorrow now, this will help with motivation & sleep

_____

_____

_____

_____

Thoughts
This is the time to write down everything that will relieve your mind. Treat this as your journal

_____

_____

_____

_____

_____

_____

_____

_____

_____

_____

_____

_____

_____

_____

_____

_____

_____

_____

_____

_____

What did today do for you?
Look back on today & reflect. Answer these questions & see what can be do one to make your life more comfortable

Name Three things that you are grateful for today:
Noting the things that we are thankful for starts & ends your day with a happy heart.

_____
_____
_____
_____

Were there any moments of sadness or stress?
And did you do anything to relieve this?

_____
_____
_____
_____

Daily aims
What did you want to achieve today? If you need to, take it into tomorrow

_____
_____
_____
_____

Self Care
It is important to spend at least 10 minutes a day to yourself, what did you do today? Meditate? Walking? Taking a warm Bath?

_____
_____
_____
_____

What are your plans for tomorrow?
Set your intentions for tomorrow now, this will help with
motivation & sleep

Thoughts
This is the time to write down everything that will relieve your
mind. Treat this as your journal

What did today do for you?
Look back on today & reflect. Answer these questions & see what can be do one to make your life more comfortable

Name Three things that you are grateful for today:
Noting the things that we are thankful for starts & ends your day with a happy heart.

_____
_____
_____
_____

Were there any moments of sadness or stress?
And did you do anything to relieve this?

_____
_____
_____
_____

Daily aims
What did you want to achieve today? If you need to, take it into tomorrow

_____
_____
_____
_____

Self Care
It is important to spend at least 10 minutes a day to yourself, what did you do today? Meditate? Walking? Taking a warm Bath?

_____
_____
_____
_____

What are your plans for tomorrow?
Set your intentions for tomorrow now, this will help with motivation & sleep

_____

_____

_____

_____

Thoughts
This is the time to write down everything that will relieve your mind. Treat this as your journal

_____

_____

_____

_____

_____

_____

_____

_____

_____

_____

_____

_____

_____

_____

_____

_____

_____

_____

_____

_____

_____

What did today do for you?
Look back on today & reflect. Answer these questions & see
what can be do one to make your life more comfortable

Name Three things that you are grateful for today:
Noting the things that we are thankful for starts & ends your day
with a happy heart.

_____

_____

_____

_____

Were there any moments of sadness or stress?
And did you do anything to relieve this?

_____

_____

_____

_____

Daily aims
What did you want to achieve today? If you need to, take it into
tomorrow

_____

_____

_____

_____

Self Care
It is important to spend at least 10 minutes a day to yourself, what
did you do today? Meditate? Walking? Taking a warm Bath?

_____

_____

_____

_____

What are your plans for tomorrow?
Set your intentions for tomorrow now, this will help with
motivation & sleep

_____

_____

_____

_____

Thoughts
This is the time to write down everything that will relieve your
mind. Treat this as your journal

_____

_____

_____

_____

_____

_____

_____

_____

_____

_____

_____

_____

_____

_____

_____

_____

_____

_____

_____

_____

_____

_____

Weekly Reflection

Now is the time to look back on your week & reflect. What worked best for you? What will you take into next week & continue with? Note below as you would a list.

What decisions have you come to, to make your day easier?

_____
_____
_____
_____

What were your highs & lows?

_____
_____
_____
_____

What would you like to tackle next week?

_____
_____
_____
_____

WELL DONE ON A SUCCESSFUL WEEK! Whether you believe it or not trying is a success in itself!

KEEP GOING! You are worth your determination

Week Eleven

What did today do for you?
Look back on today & reflect. Answer these questions & see
what can be do one to make your life more comfortable

Name Three things that you are grateful for today:
Noting the things that we are thankful for starts & ends your day
with a happy heart.

_____

_____

_____

_____

Were there any moments of sadness or stress?
And did you do anything to relieve this?

_____

_____

_____

_____

Daily aims
What did you want to achieve today? If you need to, take it into
tomorrow

_____

_____

_____

_____

Self Care
It is important to spend at least 10 minutes a day to yourself, what
did you do today? Meditate? Walking? Taking a warm Bath?

_____

_____

_____

_____

What are your plans for tomorrow?
Set your intentions for tomorrow now, this will help with motivation & sleep

_____

_____

_____

_____

Thoughts
This is the time to write down everything that will relieve your mind. Treat this as your journal

_____

_____

_____

_____

_____

_____

_____

_____

_____

_____

_____

_____

_____

_____

_____

_____

_____

_____

_____

_____

What did today do for you?

Look back on today & reflect. Answer these questions & see what can be do one to make your life more comfortable

Name Three things that you are grateful for today:

Noting the things that we are thankful for starts & ends your day with a happy heart.

_____

_____

_____

_____

Were there any moments of sadness or stress?

And did you do anything to relieve this?

_____

_____

_____

_____

Daily aims

What did you want to achieve today? If you need to, take it into tomorrow

_____

_____

_____

_____

Self Care

It is important to spend at least 10 minutes a day to yourself, what did you do today? Meditate? Walking? Taking a warm Bath?

_____

_____

_____

_____

What are your plans for tomorrow?
Set your intentions for tomorrow now, this will help with motivation & sleep

_____

_____

_____

_____

Thoughts
This is the time to write down everything that will relieve your mind. Treat this as your journal

_____

_____

_____

_____

_____

_____

_____

_____

_____

_____

_____

_____

_____

_____

_____

_____

_____

_____

_____

_____

_____

_____

What did today do for you?
Look back on today & reflect. Answer these questions & see what can be do one to make your life more comfortable

Name Three things that you are grateful for today:
Noting the things that we are thankful for starts & ends your day with a happy heart.

_____
_____
_____
_____

Were there any moments of sadness or stress?
And did you do anything to relieve this?

_____
_____
_____
_____

Daily aims
What did you want to achieve today? If you need to, take it into tomorrow

_____
_____
_____
_____

Self Care
It is important to spend at least 10 minutes a day to yourself, what did you do today? Meditate? Walking? Taking a warm Bath?

_____
_____
_____
_____

What are your plans for tomorrow?
Set your intentions for tomorrow now, this will help with
motivation & sleep

_____

_____

_____

_____

Thoughts
This is the time to write down everything that will relieve your
mind. Treat this as your journal

_____

_____

_____

_____

_____

_____

_____

_____

_____

_____

_____

_____

_____

_____

_____

_____

_____

_____

_____

_____

_____

What did today do for you?
Look back on today & reflect. Answer these questions & see what can be do one to make your life more comfortable

Name Three things that you are grateful for today:
Noting the things that we are thankful for starts & ends your day with a happy heart.

_____

_____

_____

_____

Were there any moments of sadness or stress?
And did you do anything to relieve this?

_____

_____

_____

_____

Daily aims
What did you want to achieve today? If you need to, take it into tomorrow

_____

_____

_____

_____

Self Care
It is important to spend at least 10 minutes a day to yourself, what did you do today? Meditate? Walking? Taking a warm Bath?

_____

_____

_____

_____

What are your plans for tomorrow?
Set your intentions for tomorrow now, this will help with
motivation & sleep

_____

_____

_____

_____

Thoughts
This is the time to write down everything that will relieve your
mind. Treat this as your journal

_____

_____

_____

_____

_____

_____

_____

_____

_____

_____

_____

_____

_____

_____

_____

_____

_____

_____

_____

_____

_____

_____

What did today do for you?
Look back on today & reflect. Answer these questions & see
what can be do one to make your life more comfortable

Name Three things that you are grateful for today:
Noting the things that we are thankful for starts & ends your day
with a happy heart.

_____

_____

_____

_____

Were there any moments of sadness or stress?
And did you do anything to relieve this?

_____

_____

_____

_____

Daily aims
What did you want to achieve today? If you need to, take it into
tomorrow

_____

_____

_____

_____

Self Care
It is important to spend at least 10 minutes a day to yourself, what
did you do today? Meditate? Walking? Taking a warm Bath?

_____

_____

_____

_____

What are your plans for tomorrow?
Set your intentions for tomorrow now, this will help with
motivation & sleep

_____

_____

_____

_____

Thoughts
This is the time to write down everything that will relieve your
mind. Treat this as your journal

_____

_____

_____

_____

_____

_____

_____

_____

_____

_____

_____

_____

_____

_____

_____

_____

_____

_____

_____

What did today do for you?
Look back on today & reflect. Answer these questions & see
what can be do one to make your life more comfortable

Name Three things that you are grateful for today:
Noting the things that we are thankful for starts & ends your day
with a happy heart.

_____

_____

_____

_____

Were there any moments of sadness or stress?
And did you do anything to relieve this?

_____

_____

_____

_____

Daily aims
What did you want to achieve today? If you need to, take it into
tomorrow

_____

_____

_____

_____

Self Care
It is important to spend at least 10 minutes a day to yourself, what
did you do today? Meditate? Walking? Taking a warm Bath?

_____

_____

_____

_____

What are your plans for tomorrow?
Set your intentions for tomorrow now, this will help with
motivation & sleep

_____

_____

_____

_____

Thoughts
This is the time to write down everything that will relieve your
mind. Treat this as your journal

_____

_____

_____

_____

_____

_____

_____

_____

_____

_____

_____

_____

_____

_____

_____

_____

_____

_____

_____

_____

_____

What did today do for you?

Look back on today & reflect. Answer these questions & see what can be do one to make your life more comfortable

Name Three things that you are grateful for today:

Noting the things that we are thankful for starts & ends your day with a happy heart.

_____

_____

_____

_____

Were there any moments of sadness or stress?

And did you do anything to relieve this?

_____

_____

_____

_____

Daily aims

What did you want to achieve today? If you need to, take it into tomorrow

_____

_____

_____

_____

Self Care

It is important to spend at least 10 minutes a day to yourself, what did you do today? Meditate? Walking? Taking a warm Bath?

_____

_____

_____

_____

What are your plans for tomorrow?
Set your intentions for tomorrow now, this will help with motivation & sleep

_____

_____

_____

_____

Thoughts
This is the time to write down everything that will relieve your mind. Treat this as your journal

_____

_____

_____

_____

_____

_____

_____

_____

_____

_____

_____

_____

_____

_____

_____

_____

_____

_____

_____

_____

Weekly Reflection

Now is the time to look back on your week & reflect. What worked best for you? What will you take into next week & continue with? Note below as you would a list.

What decisions have you come to, to make your day easier?

_____

_____

_____

_____

What were your highs & lows?

_____

_____

_____

_____

What would you like to tackle next week?

_____

_____

_____

_____

WELL DONE ON A SUCCESSFUL WEEK! Whether you believe it or not trying is a success in itself!

KEEP GOING! You are worth your determination

Week Twelve

What did today do for you?
Look back on today & reflect. Answer these questions & see
what can be do one to make your life more comfortable

Name Three things that you are grateful for today:
Noting the things that we are thankful for starts & ends your day
with a happy heart.

_____

_____

_____

_____

Were there any moments of sadness or stress?
And did you do anything to relieve this?

_____

_____

_____

_____

Daily aims
What did you want to achieve today? If you need to, take it into
tomorrow

_____

_____

_____

_____

Self Care
It is important to spend at least 10 minutes a day to yourself, what
did you do today? Meditate? Walking? Taking a warm Bath?

_____

_____

_____

_____

What are your plans for tomorrow?
Set your intentions for tomorrow now, this will help with motivation & sleep

_____

_____

_____

_____

Thoughts
This is the time to write down everything that will relieve your mind. Treat this as your journal

_____

_____

_____

_____

_____

_____

_____

_____

_____

_____

_____

_____

_____

_____

_____

_____

_____

_____

_____

What did today do for you?
Look back on today & reflect. Answer these questions & see
what can be do one to make your life more comfortable

Name Three things that you are grateful for today:
Noting the things that we are thankful for starts & ends your day
with a happy heart.

_____
_____
_____
_____

Were there any moments of sadness or stress?
And did you do anything to relieve this?

_____
_____
_____
_____

Daily aims
What did you want to achieve today? If you need to, take it into
tomorrow

_____
_____
_____
_____

Self Care
It is important to spend at least 10 minutes a day to yourself, what
did you do today? Meditate? Walking? Taking a warm Bath?

_____
_____
_____
_____

What are your plans for tomorrow?
Set your intentions for tomorrow now, this will help with motivation & sleep

_____

_____

_____

_____

Thoughts
This is the time to write down everything that will relieve your mind. Treat this as your journal

_____

_____

_____

_____

_____

_____

_____

_____

_____

_____

_____

_____

_____

_____

_____

_____

_____

_____

_____

_____

_____

What did today do for you?

Look back on today & reflect. Answer these questions & see
what can be do one to make your life more comfortable

Name Three things that you are grateful for today:

Noting the things that we are thankful for starts & ends your day
with a happy heart.

_____

_____

_____

_____

Were there any moments of sadness or stress?

And did you do anything to relieve this?

_____

_____

_____

_____

Daily aims

What did you want to achieve today? If you need to, take it into
tomorrow

_____

_____

_____

_____

Self Care

It is important to spend at least 10 minutes a day to yourself, what
did you do today? Meditate? Walking? Taking a warm Bath?

_____

_____

_____

_____

What are your plans for tomorrow?
Set your intentions for tomorrow now, this will help with
motivation & sleep

_____

_____

_____

_____

Thoughts
This is the time to write down everything that will relieve your
mind. Treat this as your journal

_____

_____

_____

_____

_____

_____

_____

_____

_____

_____

_____

_____

_____

_____

_____

_____

_____

_____

_____

_____

What did today do for you?

Look back on today & reflect. Answer these questions & see
what can be do one to make your life more comfortable

Name Three things that you are grateful for today:

Noting the things that we are thankful for starts & ends your day
with a happy heart.

_____

_____

_____

_____

Were there any moments of sadness or stress?

And did you do anything to relieve this?

_____

_____

_____

_____

Daily aims

What did you want to achieve today? If you need to, take it into
tomorrow

_____

_____

_____

_____

Self Care

It is important to spend at least 10 minutes a day to yourself, what
did you do today? Meditate? Walking? Taking a warm Bath?

_____

_____

_____

_____

What are your plans for tomorrow?
Set your intentions for tomorrow now, this will help with
motivation & sleep

_____

_____

_____

_____

Thoughts
This is the time to write down everything that will relieve your
mind. Treat this as your journal

_____

_____

_____

_____

_____

_____

_____

_____

_____

_____

_____

_____

_____

_____

_____

_____

_____

_____

_____

_____

What did today do for you?
Look back on today & reflect. Answer these questions & see
what can be do one to make your life more comfortable

Name Three things that you are grateful for today:
Noting the things that we are thankful for starts & ends your day
with a happy heart.

_____

_____

_____

_____

Were there any moments of sadness or stress?
And did you do anything to relieve this?

_____

_____

_____

Daily aims
What did you want to achieve today? If you need to, take it into
tomorrow

_____

_____

_____

Self Care
It is important to spend at least 10 minutes a day to yourself, what
did you do today? Meditate? Walking? Taking a warm Bath?

_____

_____

_____

What are your plans for tomorrow?
Set your intentions for tomorrow now, this will help with motivation & sleep

_____

_____

_____

_____

Thoughts
This is the time to write down everything that will relieve your mind. Treat this as your journal

What did today do for you?
Look back on today & reflect. Answer these questions & see what can be do one to make your life more comfortable

Name Three things that you are grateful for today:
Noting the things that we are thankful for starts & ends your day with a happy heart.

_____

_____

_____

_____

Were there any moments of sadness or stress?
And did you do anything to relieve this?

_____

_____

_____

_____

Daily aims
What did you want to achieve today? If you need to, take it into tomorrow

_____

_____

_____

_____

Self Care
It is important to spend at least 10 minutes a day to yourself, what did you do today? Meditate? Walking? Taking a warm Bath?

_____

_____

_____

_____

What are your plans for tomorrow?
Set your intentions for tomorrow now, this will help with
motivation & sleep

_____

_____

_____

_____

Thoughts
This is the time to write down everything that will relieve your
mind. Treat this as your journal

_____

_____

_____

_____

_____

_____

_____

_____

_____

_____

_____

_____

_____

_____

_____

_____

_____

_____

_____

_____

_____

What did today do for you?
Look back on today & reflect. Answer these questions & see what can be do one to make your life more comfortable

Name Three things that you are grateful for today:
Noting the things that we are thankful for starts & ends your day with a happy heart.

_____

_____

_____

_____

Were there any moments of sadness or stress?
And did you do anything to relieve this?

_____

_____

_____

_____

Daily aims
What did you want to achieve today? If you need to, take it into tomorrow

_____

_____

_____

_____

Self Care
It is important to spend at least 10 minutes a day to yourself, what did you do today? Meditate? Walking? Taking a warm Bath?

_____

_____

_____

_____

What are your plans for tomorrow?
Set your intentions for tomorrow now, this will help with
motivation & sleep

_____

_____

_____

_____

Thoughts
This is the time to write down everything that will relieve your
mind. Treat this as your journal

_____

_____

_____

_____

_____

_____

_____

_____

_____

_____

_____

_____

_____

_____

_____

_____

_____

_____

_____

Weekly Reflection

Now is the time to look back on your week & reflect. What
worked best for you? What will you take into next week &
continue with? Note below as you would a list.

**What decisions have you come to, to make your day
easier?**

_____

_____

_____

_____

What were your highs & lows?

_____

_____

_____

_____

What would you like to tackle next week?

_____

_____

_____

_____

WELL DONE ON A SUCCESSFUL WEEK! Whether you
believe it or not trying is a success in itself!

KEEP GOING! You are worth your determination

CONGRATULATIONS ON COMPLETING YOUR 3 MONTHS!

You've come so far & you should be so so proud. Life is full of ups and downs but being able to live your life through it will make it so much easier to cope with knowing how to manage your day.

KEEP GOING! Believe & Trust yourself!

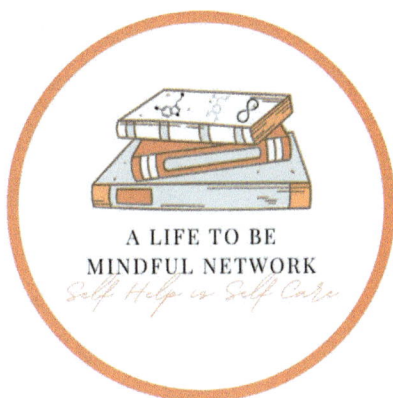

A LIFE TO BE
MINDFUL NETWORK
Self Help is Self Care